INSULIN RESISTANCE DIET COOKBOOK FOR WOMEN OVER 50

DR. JESSICA SMITH

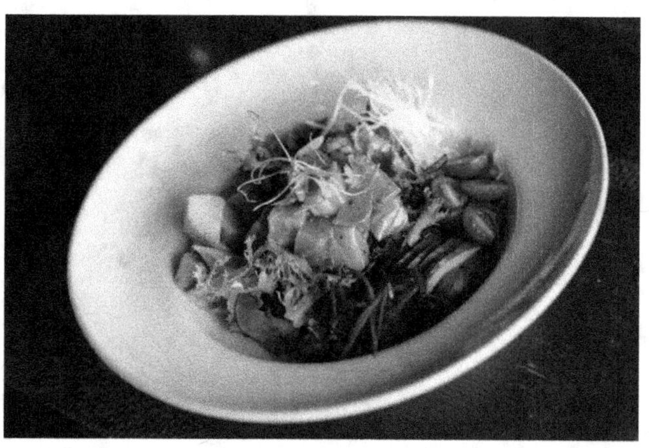

TABLE OF CONTENTS

CHAPTER ONE

How to Use this Cookbook

Understand Insulin Resistance: Educate yourself about what insulin resistance is and how it affects your body's ability to regulate blood sugar levels. This will help you grasp the importance of following a diet tailored to managing insulin resistance.

Get the Cookbook: Purchase or borrow a cookbook specifically designed for women over 50 dealing with insulin resistance. Look for one that offers a variety of tasty recipes that are low in refined carbohydrates and sugar.

Read Through the Introduction: Take the time to read through the introduction of the cookbook. Often, this section provides valuable information about insulin resistance, tips for managing it through diet, and how to use the cookbook effectively.

Review the Meal Plans: Many insulin resistance diet cookbooks offer meal plans to guide you through your journey. Review these meal plans to get an idea of what types of meals you'll be preparing and eating.

Make a Grocery List: After reviewing the meal plans, mak a grocery list of the ingredients you'll need for the recipe you want to try. Stick to the list when you go shopping t avoid buying unnecessary items.

Prep Ingredients Ahead of Time: To make mealtime easie during the week, consider prepping some ingredients ahea of time. Wash and chop vegetables, cook grains, and portio out snacks so they're ready to grab when hunger strikes.

Start Cooking: Begin trying out the recipes in th cookbook. Start with simpler recipes if you're new t cooking or short on time. As you become more comfortabl you can tackle more complex dishes.

Pay Attention to Portion Sizes: While the recipes in th cookbook are designed to be healthy for women over 50 wit insulin resistance, portion sizes still matter. Be mindful c how much you're eating and try not to overindulge, even i the food is healthy.

Listen to Your Body: Pay attention to how your bod responds to the meals you're eating. Notice if certain food make you feel more energized or if others cause you to fee luggish. Adjust your diet accordingly based on how you eel.

Stay Consistent: Consistency is key when following any liet plan. Stick to the recipes in the cookbook as much as possible, but don't be too hard on yourself if you slip up occasionally.

Remember that small changes over time can lead to big mprovements in managing insulin resistance and overall health.

Understanding Insulin Resistance Diet for Women Over 50

Understanding the Insulin Resistance Diet for women over 50 is crucial for managing a common health concern that becomes more prevalent with age.

Insulin resistance occurs when the body's cells become less responsive to insulin, a hormone that helps regulate blood sugar levels.

This resistance leads to elevated blood sugar levels, which can increase the risk of developing type 2 diabetes, heart disease, and other health issues.

Women over 50 are particularly vulnerable to insulin resistance due to hormonal changes, decreased muscle mass, and lifestyle factors.

The Insulin Resistance Diet focuses on controlling blood sugar levels by reducing the intake of refined carbohydrates and sugars while emphasizing nutrient-dense, whole foods.

This diet typically includes plenty of vegetables, lean proteins, healthy fats, and complex carbohydrates with a low glycemic index.

By choosing foods that don't cause rapid spikes in blood sugar, women over 50 can better manage their insulin levels and promote overall health.

Regular physical activity is often recommended as part of an Insulin Resistance Diet to help improve insulin sensitivity and support weight management.

Monitoring portion sizes and eating meals at regular intervals throughout the day can also help stabilize blood sugar levels.

Ultimately, understanding the Insulin Resistance Diet empowers women over 50 to take control of their health and educe the risk of developing complications associated with insulin resistance. By making informed dietary choices and adopting a healthy lifestyle, they can support their well-being and longevity.

Benefits of Insulin Resistance Diet for Women Over 50

The benefits of an Insulin Resistance Diet for women over 50 are numerous and profound, offering targeted support for managing a condition that becomes increasingly prevalent with age.

Here are several key advantages:

Blood Sugar Regulation: One of the primary benefits is the regulation of blood sugar levels. By focusing on low-glycemic index foods and reducing intake of refined carbohydrates and sugars, this diet helps stabilize blood glucose levels, preventing spikes and crashes that can contribute to insulin resistance.

Weight Management: The Insulin Resistance Diet often leads to weight loss or maintenance, which is crucial for women over 50.

Excess weight can exacerbate insulin resistance, so shedding pounds through a balanced diet can improve insulin sensitivity and overall metabolic health.

Reduced Risk of Type 2 Diabetes: By improving insulin sensitivity and promoting weight loss, this diet reduces the risk of developing type 2 diabetes, a significant concern for women over 50.

Cardiovascular Health: Following an Insulin Resistance Diet can also benefit cardiovascular health by lowering cholesterol levels, reducing blood pressure, and decreasing inflammation, thus lowering the risk of heart disease and stroke.

Increased Energy Levels: By avoiding energy crashes associated with high-glycemic foods, women over 50 may experience more consistent energy levels throughout the day, enhancing overall vitality and well-being.

Improved Hormonal Balance: Some components of the diet, such as healthy fats and lean proteins, can support hormonal balance, which is especially important for women experiencing menopause or hormonal fluctuations in their 50s.

he Insulin Resistance Diet offers a comprehensive pproach to managing insulin resistance and promoting verall health and well-being for women over 50, addressing ey concerns such as blood sugar regulation, weight anagement, and cardiovascular health.

uidelines for Insulin Resistance Diet for Vomen Over 50

uidelines for an Insulin Resistance Diet tailored to women ver 50 offer a structured approach to managing this ondition and supporting overall health. Here are key uidelines:

ocus on Whole Foods: Emphasize whole, minimally rocessed foods such as vegetables, fruits, lean proteins, uts, seeds, and whole grains. These provide essential utrients and fiber without spiking blood sugar levels.

imit Refined Carbohydrates and Sugars: Reduce intake f foods high in refined carbohydrates and sugars, such as hite bread, sugary snacks, and sweetened beverages. Opt or complex carbohydrates like quinoa, brown rice, and weet potatoes instead.

Balance Macronutrients: Aim for a balanced intake of macronutrients, including carbohydrates, proteins, and healthy fats. Incorporate sources of lean protein such as poultry, fish, tofu, and legumes, along with healthy fats like avocados, olive oil, and nuts.

Eat Regular Meals and Snacks: Spread food intake throughout the day by eating regular meals and snacks. This helps prevent large fluctuations in blood sugar levels and supports stable energy levels.

Monitor Portion Sizes: Be mindful of portion sizes to avoid overeating, which can contribute to weight gain and insulin resistance. Use smaller plates, measure servings, and pay attention to hunger and satiety cues.

Stay Hydrated: Drink plenty of water throughout the day to stay hydrated and support overall health. Limit consumption of sugary beverages and opt for water, herbal tea, or infused water instead.

Incorporate Physical Activity: Regular physical activity is essential for managing insulin resistance. Aim for a combination of aerobic exercise, strength training, and flexibility exercises to improve insulin sensitivity and support weight management.

CHAPTER TWO

: Veggie Omelette

Ingredients:

- 2 eggs
- 1/4 cup diced bell peppers (any color)
- 1/4 cup diced onions
- 1/4 cup diced tomatoes
- 1/4 cup baby spinach leaves
- Salt and pepper to taste
- 1 teaspoon olive oil

Instructions:

- In a bowl, whisk together the eggs with a pinch of salt and pepper.
- Heat olive oil in a non-stick skillet over medium heat.
- Add diced bell peppers and onions to the skillet and sauté until softened, about 2-3 minutes.

- Add diced tomatoes and baby spinach leaves to the skillet and cook for another 1-2 minutes until spinach wilts.
- Pour the whisked eggs over the vegetables in the skillet, spreading them evenly.
- Cook the omelette for 2-3 minutes until the bottom is set.
- Carefully flip the omelette and cook for an additional 1-2 minutes until cooked through.
- Slide the omelette onto a plate and fold it in half.
- Serve hot and enjoy!

Health Benefits:

- High in protein from eggs, which helps promote satiety and stabilize blood sugar levels.
- Loaded with fiber and vitamins from vegetables, supporting digestive health and providing essential nutrients.
- Low in carbohydrates, making it suitable for managing insulin resistance.

Preparation Time: 10 minutes

: Greek Yogurt Parfait

Ingredients:

- 1/2 cup plain Greek yogurt
- 1/4 cup fresh berries (such as strawberries, blueberries, or raspberries)
- 2 tablespoons chopped nuts (such as almonds or walnuts)
- 1 tablespoon unsweetened shredded coconut
- Drizzle of honey or maple syrup (optional)

Instructions:

- In a serving glass or bowl, layer half of the Greek yogurt.
- Add half of the fresh berries on top of the yogurt.
- Sprinkle half of the chopped nuts and shredded coconut over the berries.
- Repeat the layers with the remaining yogurt, berries, nuts, and coconut.
- Drizzle honey or maple syrup over the top if desired.
- Serve immediately and enjoy!

Health Benefits:

- Greek yogurt is rich in protein and probiotics, supporting gut health and promoting satiety.
- Berries are high in antioxidants and fiber, which help reduce inflammation and support digestive health.
- Nuts provide healthy fats and additional protein, aiding in blood sugar regulation and providing sustained energy.

Preparation Time: 5 minutes

3: Avocado and Egg Toast

Ingredients:

- 1 slice of whole grain bread
- 1/2 ripe avocado
- 1 egg
- Salt and pepper to taste
- Optional toppings: sliced tomatoes, sprouts, or a sprinkle of feta cheese

Instructions:

- Toast the slice of whole grain bread until golden brown.

- While the bread is toasting, mash the ripe avocado in a bowl and season with salt and pepper to taste.
- Heat a non-stick skillet over medium heat and crack the egg into the skillet.
- Cook the egg to your desired level of doneness (such as sunny-side-up or over-easy).
- Spread the mashed avocado evenly over the toasted bread.
- Carefully place the cooked egg on top of the mashed avocado.
- Add any optional toppings as desired.
- Season with additional salt and pepper if needed.
- Serve immediately and enjoy!

Health Benefits:

- Whole grain bread provides complex carbohydrates and fiber, supporting stable blood sugar levels.
- Avocado is rich in healthy fats, fiber, and vitamins, promoting heart health and providing sustained energy.

- Eggs are a good source of protein and essential nutrients, aiding in satiety and supporting muscle health.

Preparation Time: 10 minutes

4: Chia Seed Pudding

Ingredients:

- 2 tablespoons chia seeds
- 1/2 cup unsweetened almond milk (or any milk of choice)
- 1/4 teaspoon vanilla extract
- 1 teaspoon honey or maple syrup (optional)
- Fresh fruit for topping (such as sliced bananas or berries)

Instructions:

- In a bowl or jar, combine chia seeds, almond milk, vanilla extract, and honey or maple syrup if using.
- Stir well to combine.
- Cover the bowl or jar and refrigerate for at least hours or overnight, allowing the chia seeds to absorb

the liquid and thicken into a pudding-like consistency.

- Once the chia pudding has set, give it a good stir.
- Serve the chia pudding in a bowl or glass and top with fresh fruit.
- Enjoy cold!

Health Benefits:

- Chia seeds are rich in fiber, omega-3 fatty acids, and antioxidants, supporting digestive health, heart health, and inflammation reduction.
- Almond milk is low in carbohydrates and calories, making it suitable for managing blood sugar levels while providing essential nutrients like calcium and vitamin E.
- Fresh fruit adds natural sweetness and additional vitamins and minerals, enhancing the nutritional profile of the dish.

Preparation Time: 5 minutes (plus chilling time)

5: Spinach and Feta Breakfast Wrap

Ingredients:

- 1 whole wheat or low-carb tortilla
- 2 large eggs
- 1 cup fresh spinach leaves
- 2 tablespoons crumbled feta cheese
- Salt and pepper to taste
- 1 teaspoon olive oil

Instructions:

- Heat olive oil in a non-stick skillet over medium heat
- Add fresh spinach leaves to the skillet and sauté unti
  wilted, about 1-2 minutes.
- Crack the eggs into the skillet and scramble unti
  cooked through.
- Season the eggs with salt and pepper to taste.
- Warm the tortilla in the skillet or microwave for a
  few seconds to make it pliable.
- Spread the scrambled eggs evenly onto the center of
  the tortilla.
- Sprinkle crumbled feta cheese over the eggs.

- Fold the sides of the tortilla over the filling to form a wrap.
- Serve immediately and enjoy!

Health Benefits:

- Spinach is rich in vitamins, minerals, and antioxidants, supporting overall health and reducing inflammation.
- Eggs provide high-quality protein and essential nutrients, aiding in muscle maintenance and promoting satiety.
- Feta cheese adds flavor and calcium, contributing to bone health and providing essential nutrients.

Preparation Time: 10 minutes

5: Almond Flour Pancakes

Ingredients:

- 1 cup almond flour
- 2 eggs
- 1/4 cup unsweetened almond milk (or any milk of choice)
- 1 tablespoon coconut oil, melted

- 1 tablespoon honey or maple syrup (optional)
- 1/2 teaspoon baking powder
- 1/2 teaspoon vanilla extract
- Pinch of salt

Instructions:

- In a bowl, whisk together eggs, almond milk, melted coconut oil, honey or maple syrup (if using), and vanilla extract.
- Add almond flour, baking powder, and a pinch of salt to the wet ingredients.
- Stir until well combined and a smooth batter forms.
- Heat a non-stick skillet or griddle over medium heat and lightly grease with coconut oil or cooking spray.
- Pour about 1/4 cup of batter onto the skillet to form each pancake.
- Cook until bubbles form on the surface of the pancake, then flip and cook until golden brown on the other side.
- Repeat with the remaining batter.
- Serve the pancakes warm with your favorite toppings such as fresh berries or a drizzle of honey.

ealth Benefits:

- Almond flour is low in carbohydrates and rich in healthy fats, fiber, and protein, making it suitable for managing blood sugar levels and promoting satiety.
- Eggs provide additional protein and essential nutrients, supporting muscle health and satiety.
- Coconut oil adds healthy fats and flavor, while honey or maple syrup (if used) provides natural sweetness.

reparation Time: 20 minutes

Berry Protein Smoothie Bowl

ngredients:

- 1/2 cup frozen mixed berries (such as strawberries, blueberries, and raspberries)
- 1/2 ripe banana, sliced
- 1/2 cup plain Greek yogurt
- 1 scoop of protein powder (vanilla or unflavored)
- 1 tablespoon chia seeds
- 1/4 cup unsweetened almond milk (or any milk of choice)

- Toppings: sliced almonds, shredded coconut, additional berries

Instructions:

- In a blender, combine frozen mixed berries, sliced banana, Greek yogurt, protein powder, chia seeds, and almond milk.
- Blend until smooth and creamy, adding more almond milk if needed to reach desired consistency.
- Pour the smoothie into a bowl.
- Top with sliced almonds, shredded coconut, and additional berries.
- Serve immediately with a spoon and enjoy!

Health Benefits:

- Berries are rich in antioxidants and fiber, supporting heart health and digestion.
- Greek yogurt provides protein and probiotics, promoting gut health and satiety.
- Chia seeds are loaded with fiber, omega-3 fatty acids, and antioxidants, aiding in digestion and reducing inflammation.

Preparation Time: 5 minutes

Sweet Potato Breakfast Hash

Ingredients:

- 1 medium sweet potato, peeled and diced
- 1/2 red bell pepper, diced
- 1/4 red onion, diced
- 2 eggs
- 1 tablespoon olive oil
- Salt and pepper to taste
- Optional toppings: avocado slices, chopped fresh cilantro

Instructions:

- Heat olive oil in a skillet over medium heat.
- Add diced sweet potato to the skillet and cook until softened and lightly browned, about 8-10 minutes.
- Add diced red bell pepper and red onion to the skillet and cook for an additional 2-3 minutes until vegetables are tender.
- Season the hash with salt and pepper to taste.

- Create two wells in the hash and crack an egg into each well.

- Cover the skillet and cook until the eggs are cooked to your desired level of doneness, about 4-5 minutes for runny yolks.

- Once the eggs are cooked, remove the skillet from heat.

- Serve the sweet potato breakfast hash hot, topped with optional avocado slices and chopped fresh cilantro.

Health Benefits:

- Sweet potatoes are rich in fiber, vitamins, and antioxidants, supporting digestive health and reducing inflammation.

- Eggs provide high-quality protein and essential nutrients, aiding in muscle maintenance and promoting satiety.

- Bell peppers and onions add flavor and additional vitamins and minerals, enhancing the nutritional profile of the dish.

Preparation Time: 20 minutes

: Quinoa Breakfast Bowl

Ingredients:

- 1/2 cup cooked quinoa
- 1/4 cup unsweetened almond milk (or any milk of choice)
- 1/2 teaspoon ground cinnamon
- 1 tablespoon chopped nuts (such as almonds or walnuts)
- 1 tablespoon unsweetened shredded coconut
- 1/4 cup fresh berries (such as blueberries or strawberries)
- Optional: drizzle of honey or maple syrup for sweetness

Instructions:

- In a small saucepan, warm the cooked quinoa with almond milk over medium heat until heated through.
- Stir in ground cinnamon and mix well.
- Transfer the quinoa mixture to a bowl.
- Top with chopped nuts, shredded coconut, and fresh berries.

- Drizzle with honey or maple syrup if desired for added sweetness.

- Serve warm and enjoy!

Health Benefits:

- Quinoa is a nutrient-dense grain rich in protein, fiber, and essential vitamins and minerals, supporting digestive health and providing sustained energy.

- Almond milk adds creaminess and healthy fats while being low in carbohydrates, making it suitable for managing blood sugar levels.

- Nuts and berries provide additional fiber, vitamins, and antioxidants, promoting heart health and reducing inflammation.

Preparation Time: 10 minutes

10: Cottage Cheese and Fruit Bowl

Ingredients:

- 1/2 cup low-fat cottage cheese

- 1/2 cup mixed fresh fruit (such as sliced strawberries, kiwi, and pineapple)

- 1 tablespoon chopped nuts (such as almonds or pecans)
- 1 tablespoon unsweetened shredded coconut
- Optional: drizzle of honey or maple syrup for sweetness

Instructions:

- In a bowl, spoon the low-fat cottage cheese.
- Top with mixed fresh fruit, chopped nuts, and shredded coconut.
- Drizzle with honey or maple syrup if desired for added sweetness.
- Serve chilled or at room temperature and enjoy!

Health Benefits:

- Cottage cheese is rich in protein and low in carbohydrates, making it suitable for managing blood sugar levels and promoting muscle health.
- Fresh fruit provides natural sweetness, fiber, vitamins, and antioxidants, supporting overall health and reducing inflammation.

- Nuts add healthy fats and additional protein, aiding in satiety and providing sustained energy.

Preparation Time: 5 minutes

Insulin Resistance Diet Lunch Recipes for Women over 50

1: Grilled Chicken Salad

Ingredients:

- 4 oz grilled chicken breast, sliced
- 2 cups mixed salad greens (such as spinach, arugula, and kale)
- 1/2 cup cherry tomatoes, halved
- 1/4 cucumber, sliced
- 1/4 avocado, sliced
- 1 tablespoon pumpkin seeds
- 1 tablespoon crumbled feta cheese
- Balsamic vinaigrette dressing (optional)

Instructions:

- Season the chicken breast with salt and pepper and grill until cooked through.

- In a large bowl, combine the mixed salad greens, cherry tomatoes, cucumber slices, avocado slices, pumpkin seeds, and crumbled feta cheese.
- Top the salad with the sliced grilled chicken breast.
- Drizzle with balsamic vinaigrette dressing if desired.
- Toss gently to coat.
- Serve immediately and enjoy!

Health Benefits:

- Grilled chicken breast is a lean source of protein that aids in muscle maintenance and helps promote satiety.
- Mixed salad greens are rich in fiber, vitamins, and minerals, supporting digestive health and providing essential nutrients.
- Avocado provides healthy fats and fiber, promoting heart health and reducing inflammation.
- Pumpkin seeds and feta cheese add additional protein and essential nutrients, enhancing the nutritional profile of the salad.

Preparation Time: 15 minutes

2: Quinoa and Vegetable Stir-Fry

Ingredients:

- 1/2 cup cooked quinoa
- 1 cup mixed vegetables (such as bell peppers, broccoli, carrots, and snap peas), chopped
- 1 tablespoon olive oil
- 2 cloves garlic, minced
- 2 tablespoons low-sodium soy sauce or tamari
- 1 tablespoon rice vinegar
- 1 teaspoon honey or maple syrup (optional)
- Sesame seeds for garnish (optional)
- Sliced green onions for garnish (optional)

Instructions:

- Heat olive oil in a large skillet or wok over medium heat.
- Add minced garlic and sauté for 1 minute until fragrant.
- Add mixed vegetables to the skillet and stir-fry for 3-4 minutes until tender-crisp.

- In a small bowl, whisk together low-sodium soy sauce or tamari, rice vinegar, and honey or maple syrup if using.

- Add cooked quinoa to the skillet along with the sauce mixture.

- Stir-fry for an additional 2-3 minutes until everything is heated through and well combined.

- Remove from heat and garnish with sesame seeds and sliced green onions if desired.

- Serve hot and enjoy!

Health Benefits:

- Quinoa is a gluten-free whole grain rich in protein, fiber, and essential vitamins and minerals, supporting digestive health and providing sustained energy.

- Mixed vegetables are low in calories and carbohydrates but high in fiber, vitamins, and minerals, promoting overall health and reducing inflammation.

- Olive oil provides healthy fats and antioxidants, supporting heart health and reducing inflammation.

- Garlic offers immune-boosting properties and add flavor to the stir-fry.

Preparation Time: 20 minutes

3: Lentil and Vegetable Soup

Ingredients:

- 1/2 cup dried green lentils, rinsed and drained
- 4 cups low-sodium vegetable broth
- 1 cup mixed vegetables (such as carrots, celery, bel peppers, and zucchini), diced
- 1/2 onion, diced
- 2 cloves garlic, minced
- 1 teaspoon olive oil
- 1 teaspoon ground cumin
- 1/2 teaspoon ground turmeric
- Salt and pepper to taste
- Fresh parsley for garnish (optional)

Instructions:

- Heat olive oil in a large pot over medium heat.
- Add diced onion and minced garlic to the pot and sauté for 2-3 minutes until softened.

- Stir in ground cumin and ground turmeric and cook for another minute until fragrant.
- Add diced mixed vegetables to the pot and cook for 5 minutes until slightly softened.
- Pour in low-sodium vegetable broth and bring to a boil.
- Once boiling, add rinsed lentils to the pot.
- Reduce heat to low, cover, and simmer for 20-25 minutes until lentils are tender.
- Season with salt and pepper to taste.
- Ladle the soup into bowls and garnish with fresh parsley if desired.
- Serve hot and enjoy!

Health Benefits:

- Lentils are high in fiber and protein, helping stabilize blood sugar levels and promote satiety.
- Mixed vegetables provide a variety of vitamins, minerals, and antioxidants, supporting overall health and reducing inflammation.
- Olive oil adds healthy fats and flavor to the soup, supporting heart health and reducing inflammation.

- Garlic and spices like cumin and turmeric off[er]
  immune-boosting properties and add depth of flav[or]
  to the soup.

Preparation Time: 35 minutes

4: Turkey and Hummus Wrap

Ingredients:

- 4 oz sliced turkey breast
- 1 whole wheat or low-carb tortilla
- 2 tablespoons hummus
- 1/4 cup baby spinach leaves
- 1/4 cucumber, sliced
- 1/4 avocado, sliced
- Salt and pepper to taste

Instructions:

- Spread hummus evenly over the tortilla.
- Layer sliced turkey breast, baby spinach leave[s]
  cucumber slices, and avocado slices on top of th[e]
  hummus.
- Season with salt and pepper to taste.
- Roll up the tortilla tightly to form a wrap.

- Slice the wrap in half diagonally if desired.
- Serve immediately and enjoy!

Health Benefits:

- Turkey breast is a lean source of protein that aids in muscle maintenance and helps promote satiety.
- Hummus provides plant-based protein and healthy fats, supporting heart health and reducing inflammation.
- Whole wheat or low-carb tortilla adds complex carbohydrates and fiber, promoting digestive health and providing sustained energy.
- Spinach, cucumber, and avocado offer additional fiber, vitamins, and minerals, enhancing the nutritional profile of the wrap.

Preparation Time: 10 minutes

5: Salmon and Quinoa Salad

Ingredients:

- 4 oz cooked salmon fillet, flaked
- 1/2 cup cooked quinoa

- 2 cups mixed salad greens (such as spinach, arugula, and romaine)
- 1/4 cup cherry tomatoes, halved
- 1/4 cucumber, sliced
- 1/4 red onion, thinly sliced
- 1 tablespoon chopped fresh dill
- 1 tablespoon olive oil
- 1 tablespoon lemon juice
- Salt and pepper to taste

Instructions:

- In a large bowl, combine the mixed salad greens, cherry tomatoes, cucumber slices, and thinly sliced red onion.
- Add cooked quinoa to the bowl and toss to combine.
- In a small bowl, whisk together olive oil, lemon juice, chopped fresh dill, salt, and pepper to make the dressing.
- Drizzle the dressing over the salad and toss to coat evenly.
- Top the salad with flaked salmon.
- Serve immediately and enjoy!

Health Benefits:

- Salmon is rich in omega-3 fatty acids, which support heart health and reduce inflammation, and provides high-quality protein for muscle maintenance and satiety.

- Quinoa is a gluten-free whole grain packed with protein, fiber, vitamins, and minerals, supporting digestive health and providing sustained energy.

- Mixed salad greens, cherry tomatoes, cucumber, and red onion are low in calories and carbohydrates but high in fiber, vitamins, and antioxidants, promoting overall health and reducing inflammation.

- Olive oil and lemon juice provide healthy fats and flavor to the salad dressing, contributing to heart health and reducing inflammation.

Preparation Time: 20 minutes

: Eggplant and Chickpea Buddha Bowl

Ingredients:

- 1 small eggplant, diced
- 1 cup cooked chickpeas

- 1 tablespoon olive oil

- 1 teaspoon ground cumin

- 1/2 teaspoon paprika

- Salt and pepper to taste

- 2 cups cooked quinoa

- 2 cups mixed greens (such as kale or spinach)

- 1/4 cup diced red bell pepper

- 1/4 cup shredded carrots

- Tahini dressing (optional)

Instructions:

- Preheat the oven to 400°F (200°C).

- In a large bowl, toss diced eggplant with olive oil, ground cumin, paprika, salt, and pepper until evenly coated.

- Spread the seasoned eggplant in a single layer on a baking sheet lined with parchment paper.

- Roast in the preheated oven for 20-25 minutes, stirring halfway through, until the eggplant is tender and golden brown.

- In a bowl, assemble the buddha bowl by layering cooked quinoa, mixed greens, diced red bell pepper, shredded carrots, roasted eggplant, and cooked chickpeas.

- Drizzle with tahini dressing if desired.
- Serve immediately and enjoy!

ealth Benefits:

- Eggplant is low in calories and carbohydrates but rich in fiber, vitamins, and antioxidants, supporting digestive health and reducing inflammation.
- Chickpeas are high in protein and fiber, promoting satiety and stabilizing blood sugar levels.
- Quinoa provides protein, fiber, and essential nutrients, supporting digestive health and providing sustained energy.
- Mixed greens, red bell pepper, and shredded carrots offer additional fiber, vitamins, and minerals, enhancing the nutritional profile of the buddha bowl.

reparation Time: 30 minutes

Turkey and Vegetable Stir-Fry

gredients:

- 4 oz sliced turkey breast

- 1 cup mixed vegetables (such as bell pepper, broccoli, snap peas, and carrots), sliced
- 2 cloves garlic, minced
- 1 tablespoon olive oil
- 2 tablespoons low-sodium soy sauce or tamari
- 1 tablespoon rice vinegar
- 1 teaspoon honey or maple syrup (optional)
- 1/2 teaspoon grated ginger (optional)
- Sesame seeds for garnish (optional)
- Cooked brown rice or cauliflower rice for serving

Instructions:

- Heat olive oil in a large skillet or wok over medium-high heat.
- Add minced garlic to the skillet and sauté for minute until fragrant.
- Add sliced turkey breast to the skillet and stir-fry until cooked through, about 3-4 minutes.
- Add mixed vegetables to the skillet and continue to stir-fry for another 4-5 minutes until tender-crisp.

- In a small bowl, whisk together low-sodium soy sauce or tamari, rice vinegar, honey or maple syrup if using, and grated ginger if using.
- Pour the sauce mixture over the turkey and vegetables in the skillet.
- Stir well to coat everything evenly with the sauce.
- Cook for another 1-2 minutes until heated through.
- Remove from heat and garnish with sesame seeds if desired.
- Serve the turkey and vegetable stir-fry hot over cooked brown rice or cauliflower rice.

Health Benefits:

- Turkey breast provides lean protein and essential nutrients, supporting muscle maintenance and promoting satiety.
- Mixed vegetables are low in calories and carbohydrates but high in fiber, vitamins, and minerals, supporting overall health and reducing inflammation.

- Olive oil adds healthy fats and flavor to the stir-fry, contributing to heart health and reducing inflammation.

- Garlic and ginger offer immune-boosting properties and add depth of flavor to the dish.

Preparation Time: 20 minutes

8: Mediterranean Chickpea Salad

Ingredients:

- 1 can (15 oz) chickpeas, drained and rinsed
- 1 cup cherry tomatoes, halved
- 1/2 cucumber, diced
- 1/4 red onion, thinly sliced
- 1/4 cup Kalamata olives, pitted and sliced
- 2 tablespoons chopped fresh parsley
- 2 tablespoons extra-virgin olive oil
- 1 tablespoon red wine vinegar
- 1/2 teaspoon dried oregano
- Salt and pepper to taste
- Feta cheese crumbles for garnish (optional)

Instructions:

- In a large bowl, combine chickpeas, cherry tomatoes, cucumber, red onion, Kalamata olives, and chopped fresh parsley.
- In a small bowl, whisk together extra-virgin olive oil, red wine vinegar, dried oregano, salt, and pepper to make the dressing.
- Pour the dressing over the chickpea salad and toss to coat evenly.
- Garnish with feta cheese crumbles if desired.
- Serve immediately or refrigerate for 1-2 hours to allow the flavors to meld.
- Enjoy cold or at room temperature!

Health Benefits:

- Chickpeas are high in protein and fiber, promoting satiety and stabilizing blood sugar levels.
- Cherry tomatoes, cucumber, red onion, and Kalamata olives provide fiber, vitamins, and antioxidants, supporting overall health and reducing inflammation.

- Extra-virgin olive oil offers healthy fats and antioxidants, supporting heart health and reducing inflammation.
- Fresh parsley adds flavor and additional vitamins and minerals to the salad.

Preparation Time: 15 minutes

9: Tuna Salad Stuffed Avocado

Ingredients:

- 1 ripe avocado
- 1 can (5 oz) tuna, drained
- 2 tablespoons Greek yogurt
- 1 tablespoon lemon juice
- 1 stalk celery, finely chopped
- 1 tablespoon red onion, finely chopped
- Salt and pepper to taste
- Optional toppings: sliced cherry tomatoes, chopped cucumber, alfalfa sprouts

Instructions:

- Cut the ripe avocado in half and remove the pit.

- Scoop out some of the flesh from each avocado half to create a larger cavity for the filling, leaving a border around the edge.

- In a bowl, combine the drained tuna, Greek yogurt, lemon juice, chopped celery, and chopped red onion. Mix well.

- Season the tuna mixture with salt and pepper to taste.

- Spoon the tuna salad mixture into the cavity of each avocado half.

- Top with optional toppings such as sliced cherry tomatoes, chopped cucumber, or alfalfa sprouts.

- Serve immediately and enjoy!

ealth Benefits:

- Avocado provides healthy fats, fiber, and essential nutrients, promoting heart health and reducing inflammation.

- Tuna is a lean source of protein and omega-3 fatty acids, supporting muscle maintenance, heart health, and reducing inflammation.

- Greek yogurt adds creaminess and probiotics to th
  tuna salad, promoting gut health and supportin
  immune function.
- Celery and red onion provide crunch and addition:
  flavor, while also offering vitamins, minerals, an
  antioxidants.

Preparation Time: 10 minutes

10: Vegetable and Lentil Soup

Ingredients:

- 1 tablespoon olive oil
- 1/2 onion, diced
- 2 cloves garlic, minced
- 2 carrots, diced
- 2 stalks celery, diced
- 1 cup dried green lentils, rinsed and drained
- 4 cups low-sodium vegetable broth
- 1 can (14 oz) diced tomatoes
- 1 teaspoon dried thyme
- 1 teaspoon dried oregano
- Salt and pepper to taste

- Fresh parsley for garnish (optional)

Instructions:

- Heat olive oil in a large pot over medium heat.
- Add diced onion and minced garlic to the pot and sauté for 2-3 minutes until softened.
- Add diced carrots and celery to the pot and cook for another 3-4 minutes until slightly softened.
- Stir in dried green lentils, vegetable broth, diced tomatoes (with their juices), dried thyme, and dried oregano.
- Bring the soup to a boil, then reduce heat to low, cover, and simmer for 25-30 minutes until lentils are tender.
- Season the soup with salt and pepper to taste.
- Ladle the soup into bowls and garnish with fresh parsley if desired.
- Serve hot and enjoy!

Health Benefits:

- Lentils are rich in fiber and protein, helping stabilize blood sugar levels and promote satiety.

- Vegetables like carrots, celery, onion, and tomatoe provide vitamins, minerals, and antioxidants supporting overall health and reducing inflammation.
- Olive oil adds healthy fats and flavor to the soup contributing to heart health and reducing inflammation.
- Herbs like thyme and oregano offer flavor and additional antioxidants, while also providing potential immune-boosting benefits.

Preparation Time: 40 minutes

Insulin Resistance Diet Dinner Recipes for Women over 50

1: Baked Salmon with Roasted Vegetables

Ingredients:

- 2 salmon fillets (about 4-6 ounces each)
- 2 cups mixed vegetables (such as broccoli, bell peppers, zucchini, and carrots), chopped
- 2 tablespoons olive oil

- 1 teaspoon dried herbs (such as thyme, rosemary, or Italian seasoning)
- Salt and pepper to taste
- Lemon wedges for serving

Instructions:

- Preheat the oven to 400°F (200°C).
- Place the salmon fillets on a baking sheet lined with parchment paper.
- In a bowl, toss the mixed vegetables with olive oil, dried herbs, salt, and pepper until evenly coated.
- Spread the seasoned vegetables around the salmon fillets on the baking sheet.
- Bake in the preheated oven for 15-20 minutes, or until the salmon is cooked through and flakes easily with a fork, and the vegetables are tender and lightly browned.
- Remove from the oven and serve the baked salmon and roasted vegetables hot, with lemon wedges on the side.

Health Benefits:

- Salmon is rich in omega-3 fatty acids, which hav[e] anti-inflammatory properties and support hea[rt] health.
- Mixed vegetables provide fiber, vitamins, an[d] minerals, which help regulate blood sugar levels an[d] promote overall health.
- Olive oil offers healthy fats and antioxidants, whic[h] support heart health and reduce inflammation.

Preparation Time: 25 minutes

2: Turkey and Vegetable Skillet

Ingredients:

- 1 lb ground turkey
- 2 cups mixed vegetables (such as bell pepper[s] onions, carrots, and spinach), diced
- 2 cloves garlic, minced
- 1 tablespoon olive oil
- 1 teaspoon dried herbs (such as Italian seasoning o[r] thyme)
- Salt and pepper to taste

- Heat olive oil in a large skillet over medium heat.
- Add minced garlic to the skillet and sauté for 1 minute until fragrant.
- Add ground turkey to the skillet and cook, breaking it apart with a spatula, until browned and cooked through.
- Add diced mixed vegetables to the skillet and cook for 5-7 minutes, or until vegetables are tender.
- Season with dried herbs, salt, and pepper to taste, and stir well to combine.
- Remove from heat and serve the turkey and vegetable skillet hot.

Health Benefits:

- Ground turkey is a lean source of protein, which helps build and repair tissues and promotes satiety.
- Mixed vegetables provide fiber, vitamins, and minerals, which help regulate blood sugar levels and promote overall health.
- Olive oil offers healthy fats and antioxidants, which support heart health and reduce inflammation.

Preparation Time: 20 minutes

3: Quinoa-Stuffed Bell Peppers

Ingredients:

- 4 large bell peppers (any color), halved and seed removed
- 1 cup cooked quinoa
- 1 can (15 oz) black beans, drained and rinsed
- 1 cup diced tomatoes
- 1/2 cup corn kernels (fresh, canned, or frozen)
- 1/2 cup diced red onion
- 1/2 cup chopped fresh cilantro
- 1 teaspoon ground cumin
- 1/2 teaspoon chili powder
- Salt and pepper to taste
- 1/2 cup shredded cheese (cheddar, Monterey Jack, of your choice)

Instructions:

- Preheat the oven to 375°F (190°C).
- Place the halved bell peppers in a baking dish, cut side up.

- In a large bowl, combine cooked quinoa, black beans, diced tomatoes, corn kernels, diced red onion, chopped cilantro, ground cumin, chili powder, salt, and pepper. Mix well.
- Spoon the quinoa mixture evenly into each bell pepper half, pressing down lightly to pack it in.
- Cover the baking dish with aluminum foil and bake in the preheated oven for 25-30 minutes, or until the peppers are tender.
- Remove the foil and sprinkle shredded cheese over the stuffed peppers.
- Return to the oven and bake for an additional 5-10 minutes, or until the cheese is melted and bubbly.
- Remove from the oven and let cool for a few minutes before serving.

Health Benefits:

- Bell peppers are rich in vitamin C, fiber, and antioxidants, which help reduce inflammation and support immune function.

- Quinoa is a complete protein source, providing all nine essential amino acids, and is high in fiber, which helps regulate blood sugar levels and promote satiety.

- Black beans offer plant-based protein and fiber which help stabilize blood sugar levels and promote digestive health.

- Tomatoes, corn, red onion, and cilantro add flavor and additional vitamins and minerals to the dish.

Preparation Time: 45 minutes

4: Grilled Chicken and Vegetable Skewers

Ingredients:

- 2 boneless, skinless chicken breasts, cut into cubes
- 1 bell pepper (any color), cut into chunks
- 1 zucchini, sliced into rounds
- 1 red onion, cut into chunks
- 8-10 cherry tomatoes
- 1/4 cup olive oil
- 2 tablespoons balsamic vinegar
- 2 cloves garlic, minced
- 1 teaspoon dried Italian herbs (such as basil, oregano, thyme)

- Salt and pepper to taste

- Wooden or metal skewers

Instructions:

- If using wooden skewers, soak them in water for at least 30 minutes to prevent burning.

- In a bowl, whisk together olive oil, balsamic vinegar, minced garlic, dried Italian herbs, salt, and pepper to make the marinade.

- Place the chicken cubes in a shallow dish or resealable plastic bag. Pour half of the marinade over the chicken, reserving the remaining marinade for the vegetables. Toss to coat the chicken evenly. Marinate in the refrigerator for at least 30 minutes, or up to 4 hours.

- Preheat the grill to medium-high heat.

- Thread the marinated chicken cubes, bell pepper chunks, zucchini slices, red onion chunks, and cherry tomatoes onto the skewers, alternating between ingredients.

- Brush the vegetable skewers with the reserved marinade.

- Grill the skewers for 10-12 minutes, turning occasionally, until the chicken is cooked through and the vegetables are tender and slightly charred.
- Remove from the grill and let rest for a few minutes before serving.

Health Benefits:

- Chicken breast is a lean source of protein, which helps build and repair tissues and promotes satiety.
- Bell peppers, zucchini, red onion, and cherry tomatoes provide vitamins, minerals, and antioxidants, which help reduce inflammation and support overall health.
- Olive oil and balsamic vinegar offer healthy fats and flavor to the marinade, which helps promote heart health and reduce inflammation.
- Garlic and dried Italian herbs add flavor and additional antioxidants to the dish.

Preparation Time: 40 minutes

Ingredients:

- 2 boneless, skinless chicken breasts, cut into bite-sized pieces
- 2 cups mixed vegetables (such as broccoli, cauliflower, bell peppers, and carrots), chopped
- 1 cup cherry tomatoes, halved
- 1/2 onion, chopped
- 2 cloves garlic, minced
- 2 tablespoons olive oil
- 1 teaspoon dried Italian herbs (such as basil, oregano, thyme)
- Salt and pepper to taste
- 1/2 cup shredded mozzarella cheese (optional)

Instructions:

- Preheat the oven to 375°F (190°C).
- In a large mixing bowl, combine the chicken pieces, mixed vegetables, cherry tomatoes, chopped onion, minced garlic, olive oil, dried Italian herbs, salt, and pepper. Toss until everything is well coated.

- Transfer the mixture to a baking dish and spread out evenly.

- Cover the baking dish with aluminum foil and bake in the preheated oven for 25-30 minutes.

- Remove the foil and sprinkle shredded mozzarella cheese over the top (if using).

- Return the casserole to the oven and bake uncovered, for an additional 10-15 minutes, or until the chicken is cooked through and the vegetables are tender.

- Remove from the oven and let it rest for a few minutes before serving.

Health Benefits:

- Chicken breast provides lean protein, which helps support muscle health and promotes satiety.

- Mixed vegetables are low in calories and carbohydrates but high in fiber, vitamins, and minerals, which help regulate blood sugar levels and promote overall health.

- Olive oil offers healthy fats and antioxidants, which help reduce inflammation and support heart health.

- Mozzarella cheese (if using) adds calcium and protein to the dish.

Preparation Time: 45 minutes

: Lentil and Vegetable Curry

Ingredients:

- 1 cup dried green lentils, rinsed and drained
- 1 tablespoon olive oil
- 1 onion, chopped
- 2 cloves garlic, minced
- 1 tablespoon grated ginger
- 2 carrots, diced
- 1 bell pepper (any color), diced
- 1 zucchini, diced
- 1 can (14 oz) diced tomatoes
- 1 can (14 oz) coconut milk
- 2 tablespoons curry powder
- Salt and pepper to taste
- Fresh cilantro for garnish (optional)

Instructions:

- Heat olive oil in a large pot over medium heat.
- Add chopped onion, minced garlic, and grated ginger to the pot. Sauté until fragrant and onions are translucent.
- Add diced carrots, bell pepper, and zucchini to the pot. Cook for a few minutes until vegetables are slightly softened.
- Stir in the diced tomatoes (with their juices), coconut milk, curry powder, salt, and pepper.
- Add the rinsed green lentils to the pot and stir to combine.
- Bring the mixture to a boil, then reduce heat to low, cover, and simmer for 20-25 minutes, or until lentils are tender and the curry has thickened.
- Taste and adjust seasoning as needed.
- Serve the lentil and vegetable curry hot, garnished with fresh cilantro if desired. Optional: Serve with brown rice or whole grain naan bread.

Health Benefits:

- Lentils are rich in fiber and protein, which help stabilize blood sugar levels and promote satiety.
- Vegetables like carrots, bell pepper, and zucchini provide vitamins, minerals, and antioxidants, which support overall health and reduce inflammation.
- Coconut milk adds creaminess and healthy fats to the curry, which help reduce inflammation and support heart health.
- Spices like curry powder offer flavor and additional health benefits, including anti-inflammatory properties.

Preparation Time: 40 minutes

Mediterranean Chicken Skillet

Ingredients:

- 2 boneless, skinless chicken breasts, cut into strips
- 1 cup cherry tomatoes, halved
- 1/2 cup pitted Kalamata olives
- 1/4 cup diced red onion
- 2 cloves garlic, minced

- 2 tablespoons olive oil

- 1 teaspoon dried oregano

- 1/2 teaspoon dried basil

- Salt and pepper to taste

- Juice of 1 lemon

- Fresh parsley for garnish (optional)

Instructions:

- Heat olive oil in a large skillet over medium-high heat.

- Add minced garlic to the skillet and sauté for 1 minute until fragrant.

- Add chicken breast strips to the skillet and cook until browned on all sides and cooked through, about 6-8 minutes.

- Add halved cherry tomatoes, pitted Kalamata olives, diced red onion, dried oregano, dried basil, salt, and pepper to the skillet. Stir to combine.

- Cook for an additional 2-3 minutes, until the tomatoes are softened and the flavors have melded together.

- Squeeze lemon juice over the chicken and Mediterranean mixture, and toss to combine.
- Remove from heat and garnish with fresh parsley if desired.
- Serve hot and enjoy!

Health Benefits:

- Chicken breast provides lean protein, which helps support muscle health and promotes satiety.
- Cherry tomatoes and red onion offer vitamins, minerals, and antioxidants, which support overall health and reduce inflammation.
- Kalamata olives provide healthy fats and antioxidants, which support heart health and reduce inflammation.
- Olive oil adds healthy fats and flavor to the skillet, which helps reduce inflammation and supports heart health.

Preparation Time: 20 minutes

8: Cauliflower Fried Rice

Ingredients:

- 1 medium head cauliflower, grated or riced
- 2 tablespoons olive oil
- 2 cloves garlic, minced
- 1/2 cup diced carrots
- 1/2 cup frozen peas
- 2 green onions, thinly sliced
- 2 eggs, beaten
- 2 tablespoons low-sodium soy sauce or tamari
- 1 teaspoon sesame oil
- Salt and pepper to taste
- Sesame seeds for garnish (optional)

Instructions:

- Heat olive oil in a large skillet or wok over medium heat.
- Add minced garlic to the skillet and sauté for 1 minute until fragrant.
- Add diced carrots and frozen peas to the skillet and cook for 3-4 minutes until slightly softened.

- Push the vegetables to one side of the skillet and pour beaten eggs into the empty side.

- Scramble the eggs until cooked through, then mix them with the vegetables.

- Add grated or riced cauliflower to the skillet and stir to combine.

- Drizzle low-sodium soy sauce or tamari and sesame oil over the cauliflower mixture. Stir well to evenly distribute the sauces.

- Cook for an additional 3-4 minutes, stirring occasionally, until the cauliflower is tender and heated through.

- Season with salt and pepper to taste.

- Remove from heat and garnish with sesame seeds if desired.

- Serve hot and enjoy!

Health Benefits:

- Cauliflower is low in calories and carbohydrates but high in fiber and antioxidants, which support digestion and reduce inflammation.

- Carrots and peas provide vitamins, minerals, and antioxidants, which support overall health and reduce inflammation.

- Eggs offer high-quality protein and essential nutrients, which support muscle health and promote satiety.

- Olive oil and sesame oil provide healthy fats and flavor to the dish, which help reduce inflammation and support heart health.

Preparation Time: 25 minutes

9: Shrimp and Vegetable Stir-Fry

Ingredients:

- 1 lb large shrimp, peeled and deveined

- 2 cups mixed vegetables (such as broccoli, bell peppers, snap peas, and carrots), sliced

- 2 cloves garlic, minced

- 1 tablespoon olive oil

- 2 tablespoons low-sodium soy sauce or tamari

- 1 tablespoon rice vinegar

- 1 teaspoon honey or maple syrup (optional)

- 1/2 teaspoon grated ginger (optional)

- Sesame seeds for garnish (optional)

- Cooked brown rice or cauliflower rice for serving

Instructions:

- In a large skillet or wok, heat olive oil over medium-high heat.

- Add minced garlic to the skillet and sauté for 1 minute until fragrant.

- Add sliced mixed vegetables to the skillet and stir-fry for 3-4 minutes until slightly softened.

- Push the vegetables to one side of the skillet and add shrimp to the other side.

- Cook the shrimp for 2-3 minutes on each side until pink and cooked through.

- In a small bowl, whisk together low-sodium soy sauce or tamari, rice vinegar, honey or maple syrup if using, and grated ginger if using.

- Pour the sauce mixture over the shrimp and vegetables in the skillet.

- Stir well to coat everything evenly with the sauce.

- Cook for another 1-2 minutes until heated through.

- Remove from heat and garnish with sesame seeds if
  desired.
- Serve the shrimp and vegetable stir-fry hot over
  cooked brown rice or cauliflower rice.

Health Benefits:

- Shrimp is low in calories and saturated fat but high
  in protein, which supports muscle health and
  promotes satiety.
- Mixed vegetables provide fiber, vitamins, and
  minerals, which help regulate blood sugar levels and
  support overall health.
- Olive oil offers healthy fats and antioxidants, which
  help reduce inflammation and support heart health.
- Garlic and ginger offer immune-boosting properties
  and add depth of flavor to the dish.

Preparation Time: 20 minutes

10: Turkey and Spinach Stuffed Portobello Mushrooms

Ingredients:

- 4 large portobello mushrooms, stems removed

- 1 lb ground turkey

- 2 cups fresh spinach leaves, chopped

- 1/2 onion, diced

- 2 cloves garlic, minced

- 1 tablespoon olive oil

- 1 teaspoon dried Italian herbs (such as basil, oregano, thyme)

- Salt and pepper to taste

- 1/2 cup shredded mozzarella cheese (optional)

- Fresh parsley for garnish (optional)

Instructions:

- Preheat the oven to 375°F (190°C). Line a baking sheet with parchment paper.

- Place portobello mushrooms on the prepared baking sheet, gill side up.

- In a large skillet, heat olive oil over medium heat.

- Add diced onion and minced garlic to the skillet and sauté for 2-3 minutes until softened.

- Add ground turkey to the skillet and cook until browned and cooked through, breaking it apart with a spatula.

- Stir in chopped spinach leaves and dried Italian herbs. Cook for another 2-3 minutes until spinach wilted.

- Season the turkey mixture with salt and pepper to taste.

- Spoon the turkey and spinach mixture evenly into each portobello mushroom cap.

- If using, sprinkle shredded mozzarella cheese over the top of each stuffed mushroom.

- Bake in the preheated oven for 15-20 minutes, or until the mushrooms are tender and the cheese melted and bubbly.

- Remove from the oven and garnish with fresh parsley if desired.

- Serve the stuffed portobello mushrooms hot.

Health Benefits:

- Portobello mushrooms are low in calories and carbohydrates but high in fiber and antioxidants which support digestion and reduce inflammation.

- Turkey provides lean protein, which helps support muscle health and promotes satiety.

- Spinach offers vitamins, minerals, and antioxidants, which support overall health and reduce inflammation.

- Mozzarella cheese (optional) adds calcium and protein to the dish.

Preparation Time: 30 minutes

Insulin Resistance Diet Snacks Recipes for Women over 50

: Greek Yogurt Parfait

Ingredients:

- 1 cup Greek yogurt (plain, unsweetened)
- 1/2 cup mixed berries (such as strawberries, blueberries, raspberries)
- 1/4 cup granola (choose a low-sugar or homemade option)
- 1 tablespoon honey (optional)
- 1 tablespoon chopped nuts (such as almonds, walnuts) for topping (optional)
- Instructions:

- In a serving glass or bowl, layer Greek yogurt, mixed berries, and granola.

- Drizzle honey over the top if desired.

- Repeat the layers until the glass or bowl is filled finishing with a layer of granola on top.

- Sprinkle chopped nuts over the granola for added crunch and nutrition.

- Serve immediately and enjoy!

Health Benefits:

- Greek yogurt is rich in protein and probiotics, which promote digestive health and support immune function.

- Mixed berries provide antioxidants, fiber, and vitamins, which help reduce inflammation and support overall health.

- Granola offers fiber and healthy fats for sustained energy, but be mindful of added sugars and choose a low-sugar option or make your own.

- Honey adds natural sweetness, but use sparingly to control sugar intake.

Preparation Time: 5 minutes

: Veggie Sticks with Hummus

ngredients:

- Assorted vegetable sticks (such as carrot, cucumber, bell pepper, celery)
- 1/2 cup hummus (store-bought or homemade)
- Optional: lemon juice, olive oil, paprika, or cumin for seasoning hummus

nstructions:

- Wash and cut assorted vegetables into sticks.
- If making homemade hummus, blend chickpeas, tahini, lemon juice, garlic, olive oil, salt, and any additional seasonings until smooth. Adjust consistency with water as needed.
- Serve vegetable sticks with hummus for dipping.
- Optional: Drizzle hummus with a little olive oil and sprinkle with paprika, cumin, or a squeeze of lemon juice for extra flavor.
- Enjoy as a healthy and satisfying snack!

Health Benefits:

- Assorted vegetable sticks provide fiber, vitamins and minerals, which help regulate blood sugar level and promote overall health.

- Hummus offers plant-based protein, fiber, and healthy fats, which support satiety and heart health.

- Optional seasonings like paprika, cumin, and lemon juice add flavor without extra calories or sugar.

Preparation Time: 10 minutes

3: Avocado and Tomato Salsa

Ingredients:

- 1 ripe avocado, diced
- 1 large tomato, diced
- 1/4 cup red onion, finely chopped
- 1 tablespoon fresh cilantro, chopped
- Juice of 1 lime
- Salt and pepper to taste
- Optional: jalapeño, diced, for added heat

Instructions:

- In a mixing bowl, combine diced avocado, tomato, red onion, and chopped cilantro.
- Squeeze lime juice over the mixture and gently toss to combine.
- Season with salt and pepper to taste.
- If desired, add diced jalapeño for extra heat.
- Serve immediately with whole grain crackers or vegetable sticks.
- Enjoy this refreshing and nutritious snack!

Health Benefits:

- Avocado provides healthy fats, fiber, and essential nutrients, promoting heart health and reducing inflammation.
- Tomatoes are rich in antioxidants, vitamins, and minerals, which support overall health and reduce inflammation.
- Red onion offers flavor and additional antioxidants, while also providing potential immune-boosting benefits.

- Lime juice adds a tangy flavor and provides vitamin C, which supports immune function.

Preparation Time: 10 minutes

4: Cottage Cheese and Apple Slices

Ingredients:

- 1/2 cup low-fat cottage cheese
- 1 medium apple, sliced
- 1 tablespoon almond butter or peanut butter
- Optional toppings: cinnamon, honey, chopped nuts

Instructions:

- Place low-fat cottage cheese in a serving bowl.
- Slice the apple and arrange the slices alongside the cottage cheese.
- Drizzle almond butter or peanut butter over the apple slices.
- Sprinkle with optional toppings such as cinnamon, honey, or chopped nuts.
- Enjoy this protein-packed and satisfying snack!

Health Benefits:

- Cottage cheese is high in protein and calcium, which supports muscle health and bone strength.
- Apples provide fiber, vitamins, and antioxidants, which help regulate blood sugar levels and promote overall health.
- Almond butter or peanut butter offers healthy fats and additional protein, which helps promote satiety and stabilize blood sugar levels.
- Optional toppings like cinnamon, honey, or chopped nuts add flavor and extra nutrients without excess sugar or calories.

Preparation Time: 5 minutes

: Cucumber and Hummus Bites

Ingredients:

- 1 large cucumber
- 1/2 cup hummus (store-bought or homemade)
- Optional toppings: cherry tomatoes, sliced olives, fresh herbs

Instructions:

- Wash the cucumber and cut it into thick rounds.
- Using a small spoon or melon baller, scoop out a small portion from the center of each cucumber round to create a hollow.
- Fill each cucumber round with a dollop of hummus.
- Top with optional toppings such as cherry tomatoes, sliced olives, or fresh herbs.
- Arrange the cucumber and hummus bites on a serving platter.
- Serve immediately and enjoy this refreshing and nutritious snack!

Health Benefits:

- Cucumber is low in calories and high in water content, making it hydrating and refreshing.
- Hummus provides plant-based protein, fiber, and healthy fats, which promote satiety and stabilize blood sugar levels.
- Optional toppings like cherry tomatoes, sliced olives, or fresh herbs add flavor, vitamins, and minerals without excess calories or sugar.

reparation Time: 10 minutes

: Almond Berry Smoothie

ngredients:

- 1 cup unsweetened almond milk
- 1/2 cup frozen mixed berries (such as strawberries, blueberries, raspberries)
- 1/2 ripe banana
- 2 tablespoons almond butter
- 1 tablespoon chia seeds
- Optional: honey or maple syrup to taste

nstructions:

- In a blender, combine unsweetened almond milk, frozen mixed berries, ripe banana, almond butter, and chia seeds.
- If desired, add a drizzle of honey or maple syrup for sweetness.
- Blend until smooth and creamy.
- Pour the smoothie into a glass.
- Garnish with additional berries or a sprinkle of chia seeds if desired.

- Serve immediately and enjoy this delicious and filling smoothie!

Health Benefits:

- Almond milk is low in calories and carbohydrates, making it a suitable base for a low-glycemic smoothie.
- Mixed berries are rich in antioxidants, fiber, and vitamins, which help regulate blood sugar levels and support overall health.
- Banana adds natural sweetness and provides potassium, which supports heart health and muscle function.
- Almond butter offers healthy fats and protein, which help promote satiety and stabilize blood sugar levels.
- Chia seeds are high in fiber and omega-3 fatty acids, which support digestive health and reduce inflammation.

Preparation Time: 5 minutes

Edamame and Veggie Dip

Ingredients:

- 1 cup shelled edamame (frozen or fresh)
- 1/4 cup plain Greek yogurt
- 1 tablespoon lemon juice
- 1 clove garlic, minced
- 1 tablespoon fresh parsley, chopped
- Salt and pepper to taste
- Assorted vegetable sticks (such as carrot, cucumber, bell pepper)

Instructions:

- Cook the shelled edamame according to package instructions, then drain and let cool.
- In a food processor, combine cooked edamame, plain Greek yogurt, lemon juice, minced garlic, chopped parsley, salt, and pepper.
- Blend until smooth and creamy, adding a little water if needed to reach the desired consistency.
- Transfer the dip to a serving bowl.
- Arrange assorted vegetable sticks on a platter.

- Serve the edamame dip alongside the vegetab[le] sticks.

- Enjoy this protein-packed and flavorful snack!

Health Benefits:

- Edamame is rich in plant-based protein, fiber, an[d] antioxidants, which support muscle health an[d] reduce inflammation.

- Greek yogurt provides additional protein an[d] probiotics, which promote digestive health an[d] support immune function.

- Lemon juice adds a refreshing flavor and provide[s] vitamin C, which supports immune function.

- Assorted vegetable sticks offer fiber, vitamins, an[d] minerals, which help regulate blood sugar levels an[d] promote overall health.

Preparation Time: 15 minutes

8: Tuna Salad Lettuce Wraps

Ingredients:

- 1 can (5 oz) tuna in water, drained
- 2 tablespoons plain Greek yogurt

- 1 tablespoon Dijon mustard

- 1/4 cup diced celery

- 1/4 cup diced red onion

- 1 tablespoon fresh dill, chopped

- Salt and pepper to taste

- 4 large lettuce leaves (such as butter lettuce or romaine)

Instructions:

- In a mixing bowl, combine drained tuna, plain Greek yogurt, Dijon mustard, diced celery, diced red onion, chopped fresh dill, salt, and pepper.

- Stir until well combined.

- Place a spoonful of the tuna salad mixture onto each lettuce leaf.

- Roll up the lettuce leaves to create wraps.

- Serve immediately and enjoy these light and protein-rich lettuce wraps!

Health Benefits:

- Tuna is a lean source of protein, which helps support muscle health and promote satiety.

- Greek yogurt provides additional protein and probiotics, which promote digestive health and support immune function.

- Celery and red onion offer fiber, vitamins, and minerals, which help regulate blood sugar levels and support overall health.

- Lettuce leaves provide a low-calorie and hydrating alternative to traditional wraps or bread.

Preparation Time: 10 minutes

9: Roasted Chickpeas

Ingredients:

- 1 can (15 oz) chickpeas (garbanzo beans), drained and rinsed

- 1 tablespoon olive oil

- 1 teaspoon ground cumin

- 1/2 teaspoon smoked paprika

- 1/2 teaspoon garlic powder

- 1/2 teaspoon salt

- 1/4 teaspoon black pepper

Instructions:

- Preheat the oven to 400°F (200°C) and line a baking sheet with parchment paper.
- Pat the chickpeas dry with a paper towel to remove excess moisture.
- In a bowl, toss the chickpeas with olive oil, ground cumin, smoked paprika, garlic powder, salt, and black pepper until evenly coated.
- Spread the seasoned chickpeas in a single layer on the prepared baking sheet.
- Bake in the preheated oven for 25-30 minutes, shaking the pan halfway through, until the chickpeas are crispy and golden brown.
- Remove from the oven and let cool slightly before serving.
- Enjoy these crunchy roasted chickpeas as a healthy and satisfying snack!

Health Benefits:

- Chickpeas are rich in protein and fiber, which help regulate blood sugar levels and promote satiety.

- Olive oil provides healthy fats and antioxidants, which support heart health and reduce inflammation.

- Spices like cumin, paprika, and garlic powder add flavor and additional health benefits, including anti-inflammatory properties.

Preparation Time: 35 minutes

10: Kale Chips

Ingredients:

- 1 bunch kale, stems removed and torn into bite-sized pieces

- 1 tablespoon olive oil

- 1 tablespoon nutritional yeast (optional)

- 1/2 teaspoon garlic powder

- 1/2 teaspoon smoked paprika

- 1/4 teaspoon salt

Instructions:

- Preheat the oven to 300°F (150°C) and line a baking sheet with parchment paper.

- In a large bowl, massage the torn kale leaves with olive oil until evenly coated.

- Sprinkle nutritional yeast (if using), garlic powder, smoked paprika, and salt over the kale leaves. Toss to coat.

- Spread the seasoned kale leaves in a single layer on the prepared baking sheet.

- Bake in the preheated oven for 20-25 minutes, or until the kale is crispy but not burnt, checking and flipping halfway through.

- Remove from the oven and let cool slightly before serving.

- Enjoy these crunchy kale chips as a nutritious and delicious snack!

Health Benefits:

- Kale is packed with vitamins, minerals, and antioxidants, which support overall health and reduce inflammation.

- Olive oil provides healthy fats and antioxidants, which support heart health and reduce inflammation.

- Spices like garlic powder and smoked paprika add flavor and additional health benefits, including anti-inflammatory properties.

Preparation Time: 30 minutes

CONCLUSION

In conclusion, the Insulin Resistance Diet Cookbook for Women Over 50 serves as a comprehensive guide and invaluable resource for those navigating the complexities of managing insulin resistance.

By embracing a balanced and nutritious approach to eating, this cookbook empowers women over 50 to take charge of their health and well-being.

Through a collection of delicious and easy-to-prepare recipes, this cookbook demonstrates that managing insulin resistance doesn't mean sacrificing flavor or satisfaction.

Instead, it opens the door to a world of culinary possibilities that prioritize wholesome ingredients and mindful eating habits.

From energizing breakfasts to satisfying dinners and everything in between, each recipe is thoughtfully crafted to support stable blood sugar levels, promote satiety, and nourish the body with essential nutrients.

With a focus on whole foods, lean proteins, healthy fats, and fiber-rich carbohydrates, these recipes provide a roadmap to better health and vitality.

Moreover, this cookbook goes beyond just recipes, offering valuable insights into the principles of the Insulin Resistance Diet and practical tips for success.

It empowers women over 50 to make informed choices about their diet and lifestyle, ultimately leading to improved health outcomes and a greater sense of well-being.

The Insulin Resistance Diet Cookbook for Women Over 50 is not just a cookbook but a trusted companion on the journey to better health.

It inspires confidence in the kitchen, fosters a deeper understanding of insulin resistance, and lays the foundation for a lifetime of healthy eating habits.

With this cookbook in hand, women over 50 can embrace a delicious and fulfilling approach to managing insulin resistance and thriving at every stage of life.